VASCULITIS
DIET COOKBOOK
FOR BEGINNERS

A SIMPLE GUIDE WITH QUICK AND HEALTHY ANTI-INFLAMMATORY RECIPES FOR HEALING AND MANAGING SYMPTOMS FOR OPTIMAL WELL-BEING

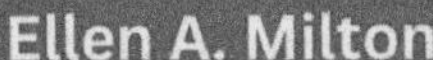

Ellen A. Milton

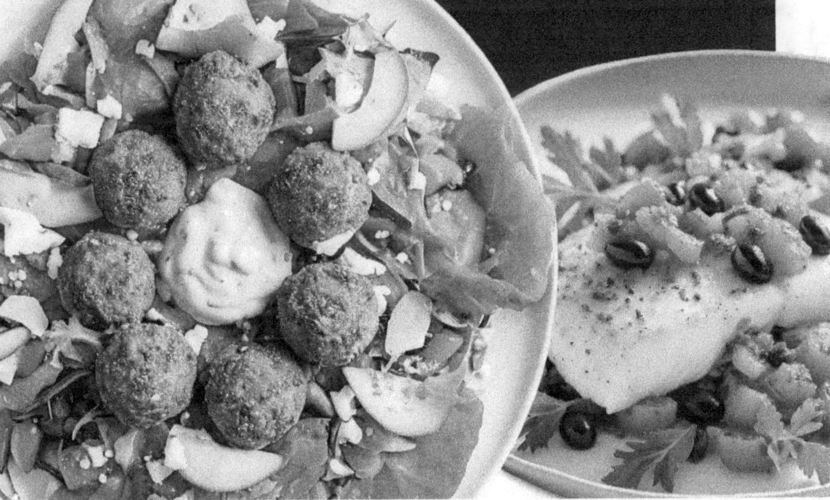

This book is for informational purposes only. The content is not intended to be a substitute for professional medical advice, diagnosis, or treatment. Always seek the advice of your physician or other qualified healthcare provider with any questions you may have regarding a medical condition.

Table Of Content

Introduction

I understand that dealing with vasculitis may be daunting. The inflammation, pain, and uncertainty are a lot to deal with on top of daily living. But I want you to know that there is hope, and that right diet may make a huge difference in your path to healing and wellbeing.

Vasculitis is a complicated disorder that affects your blood vessels, causing them to become inflamed and possibly leading to a variety of unpleasant side effects. But the good news is that by fueling your body with the correct nutrients, you can help reduce inflammation, strengthen your immune system, and regain control of your health.

That's why i created this cookbook: a simple yet comprehensive guide to navigating the vasculitis diet. My objective is to provide you with the information and skills you need to take charge of your health, one tasty and nutritious meal at a time.

These book will provide you a thorough explanation of the many varieties of vasculitis, typical symptoms, and how the appropriate foods may help you find relief. We'll go into the essential nutrients your body need, as well as the foods you should prioritize and those to restrict or avoid.

However, this is not just a dry, theoretical approach. I've also included a 2-week meal plan with meals for breakfast, lunch, dinner, snacks, and desserts. These are fast, healthful, and, most importantly, quite tasty. Because I believe that healing should not entail giving up the pleasure of eating.

So, I invite you to dive in, read these pages, and find a whole new universe of possibilities for controlling your vasculitis. With the correct information and recipes, you can regain control of your health and begin to feel better.

Chapter 1

Understanding Vasculitis and Nutrition

I understand how confusing the world of vasculitis can be, with so many distinct forms and symptoms. However, recognizing this illness and how proper diet may assist manage it is the first step toward reclaiming control of your health.

1.1 Overview of the different types of vasculitis

Understanding vasculitis requires acknowledging that it is not a single syndrome, but rather a varied family of conditions. Each variety of vasculitis is distinct, with its own set of symptoms, causes, and possible consequences for the body. Let us take a deeper look at the many manifestations of this complicated illness.

1. Large-Vessel Vasculitis: This category includes illnesses such as giant cell arteritis and Takayasu's arteritis, which principally affect the body's biggest arteries, the aorta and its major branches. If not treated, this types of vasculitis may cause limited blood flow, aneurysms, and possibly life-threatening consequences.

2. Medium-Vessel Vasculitis: includes polyarteritis nodosa and Kawasaki illness. These forms of vasculitis typically affect the medium-sized arteries, which may cause organ damage, tissue death, and an increased risk of cardiac problems.

3. Small-Vessel Vasculitis: This category includes a variety of illnesses, including ANCA-associated vasculitis (granulomatosis with polyangiitis and microscopic polyangiitis) and immune complex vasculitis (IgA vasculitis and cryoglobulinemia). These types of vasculitis often attack smaller blood vessels, causing inflammation, bleeding, and possible organ damage.

4. Variable-Vessel Vasculitis: This group includes Behçet's disease and Cogan's syndrome, which damage blood arteries of variable sizes throughout the body. This flexibility may make certain types of vasculitis difficult to control and cure.

5. Single-Organ Vasculitis: In certain circumstances, vasculitis affects just one organ or tissue, such as the skin (cutaneous vasculitis) or the central nervous system. Although less prevalent, these localized types of vasculitis may have a substantial effect on your health and quality of life.

Remember that knowledge is power, and the more you learn about the complexities of vasculitis, the more prepared you will be to navigate this path to good health. Let's continue our journey and discover how nutrition may help you manage your symptoms and improve your overall health.

1.2 Common Symptoms, Causes, and Risk Factors—and How Diet Can Help Manage Them

As we learn more about vasculitis, it's important to look at the typical symptoms, causes, and risk factors linked with this complicated disorder. More significantly, I'd want to show you how a well-planned diet may help you manage these issues and improve your overall health.

1. Fatigue and Muscle Weakness: Vasculitis may reduce blood supply to numerous regions of the body, including the muscles, resulting in a deep sensation of fatigue and weakness. A diet high in nutrient-dense foods that promote energy generation, such as complex carbs, lean proteins, and healthy fats, may help alleviate this distressing condition. Whole grains, leafy greens, and fatty fish may give the energy your body needs to operate properly.

2. Joint and Muscle Pain: Inflammation, which is characteristic of vasculitis, may cause substantial pain in the joints and muscles. Incorporating anti-inflammatory foods like turmeric and ginger, as well as omega-3-rich foods like walnuts and chia seeds, will help decrease inflammation and soothe this distressing condition. Additionally, staying hydrated and eating foods strong in antioxidants, such as berries and bell peppers, might help your body's natural healing processes.

3. Skin Rashes and Lesions: Vasculitis may cause a variety of skin concerns, including rashes, hives, and even open sores or lesions. A diet high in skin-nourishing elements, such as vitamin C, zinc, and healthy fats, may help to build the skin's barrier and encourage healing. Citrus foods, almonds, and avocados are especially effective in treating these skin issues.

4. Organ Damage: Depending on the kind of vasculitis, the inflammation may affect essential organs including the kidneys, lungs, or heart. A diet rich in antioxidants, anti-inflammatory compounds, and minerals such as omega-3 fatty acids may help reduce the risk of organ damage and promote healthy function. Leafy vegetables, fatty fish, and berries are all wonderful options in this regard.

5. Neurological Symptoms: In certain situations, vasculitis may damage blood vessels in the brain, resulting in neurological symptoms such as headaches, dizziness, and cognitive impairment. Incorporating brain-boosting foods like nuts, seeds, and leafy greens will assist promote neurological health and perhaps reduce these distressing symptoms.

6. Digestive Issues: Vasculitis may sometimes affect the digestive tract, resulting in stomach discomfort, nausea, and even gastrointestinal bleeding. A diet rich in gut-friendly foods, such as fermented vegetables, high-fiber whole grains, and probiotic-rich yogurt, may maintain a healthy gut microbiome and reduce digestive issues.

Understanding the many symptoms, causes, and risk factors linked with vasculitis allows you to take proactive steps to alleviate them using the power of nutrition. By combining the correct foods and dietary choices, you may help manage your symptoms, support your body's natural healing processes, and, eventually, improve your overall health.

Chapter 2

Understanding the Vasculitis Diet

2.1 Key nutrients and dietary considerations for vasculitis

As someone living with vasculitis, you must be particularly mindful of the nutrition your body needs to operate properly. Allow me to break it down for you:

1. Anti-inflammatory Nutrients: Because vasculitis is an inflammatory disorder, it's important to eat nutrients that may help lower inflammation in the body. This contains healthy fats like omega-3 fatty acids (found in fatty fish, walnuts, and flaxseeds), antioxidants (berries, leafy greens, bell peppers), and anti-inflammatory spices like turmeric and ginger.

2. Protein: Maintaining a sufficient protein intake is critical for tissue repair, immunological function, and general healing. Choose lean protein sources such as poultry, fish, eggs, legumes, and plant-based proteins like tofu or tempeh. These nutrient-dense alternatives will provide your body the building blocks it needs to counteract the symptoms of vasculitis.

3. Hydration: Staying hydrated is essential for eliminating toxins, decreasing inflammation, and maintaining organ function. Aim for at least 8 glasses of water or other fluids each day, such as herbal tea and broth-based soup. Keeping your body hydrated might help relieve fatigue and joint discomfort.

4. Fiber: Fiber-rich foods such as whole grains, fruits, vegetables, and legumes are not only beneficial to digestive health, but they also aid in blood sugar regulation and immunological function. Incorporating these nutrient-dense foods may deliver an abundance of vitamins, minerals, and antioxidants.

5. Probiotics: The gut plays an important role in immune function, and vasculitis may upset the delicate balance of gut flora. Consuming probiotic-rich foods such as yogurt, kefir, and fermented vegetables may help restore gut health and boost your body's natural defense mechanisms.

6. Vitamin C: This potent antioxidant is required for immunological function and collagen formation, both of which are critical for maintaining healthy blood vessels. Citrus fruits, bell peppers, broccoli, and leafy greens are all rich in vitamin C.

7. Vitamin D: Many people with vasculitis have low levels of vitamin D, which is essential for bone health, immunological function, and inflammation control. Sunlight, fatty fish, and fortified meals may help you maintain healthy vitamin D levels.

2.2 Foods to focus on

Focusing on the appropriate meals may help decrease inflammation, improve your immune system, and give the nutrients your body needs.

Let's get into the foods you'll want to try:

1. Fatty Fish: Salmon, mackerel, sardines, and tuna contain omega-3 fatty acids, which are powerful anti-inflammatory agents. These good fats may help to reduce the underlying inflammation that typically accompanies vasculitis, alleviating symptoms such as joint discomfort and skin irritation.

2. Leafy Greens: Kale, spinach, arugula, and collard greens include critical vitamins, minerals, and antioxidants that promote general health. These greens' high phytonutrient content may aid in immune system regulation and inflammation reduction throughout the body.

3. Berries: Blueberries, raspberries, blackberries, and strawberries are high in antioxidants and anti-inflammatory chemicals. Incorporating these colorful fruits into your diet will help preserve your cells and support your body's natural healing processes.

4. Turmeric: This colorful spice includes curcumin, a powerful chemical that has been demonstrated to have potent anti-inflammatory benefits. Adding turmeric to your meals, either as a spice or as a supplement, may help reduce the inflammation caused by vasculitis.

5. Garlic and onions: These tasty alliums are high in sulfur-containing chemicals, which have been shown to have anti-inflammatory and immune-boosting properties. Incorporating them into your cooking may benefit your overall health.

6. Nuts and Seeds: Almonds, walnuts, chia seeds, and flaxseeds are high in healthy fats, fiber, vitamins, and minerals. These healthful foods include anti-inflammatory omega-3s, which may help reduce inflammation and boost your body's natural defenses.

7. Bone Broth: Drinking homemade bone broth might give several advantages for those with vasculitis. Bone broth contains collagen, gelatin, and amino acids, which may aid with immune function, gastrointestinal health, and tissue repair.

8. Probiotic-Rich Foods: Yogurt, kefir, sauerkraut, and kimchi are all high in good gut bacteria that may help regulate your immune system and decrease inflammation. Nourishing your gut microbiota may have far-reaching benefits for your overall health.

Focusing on these nutrient-dense, anti-inflammatory foods will offer your body with the necessary building blocks to manage your vasculitis symptoms and support your road to maximum health. Remember, persistence and experimentation are essential; listen to your body and discover the exact combination of meals that work best for you.

2.3 Foods to limit or avoid

Let's look at the meals you may like to restrict or avoid:

1. Processed and fried foods: These are abundant in harmful fats, processed carbs, and additives, all of which may lead to inflammation. Processed meats, fast food, and fried snacks should be consumed in moderation or avoided altogether.

2. Refined Carbohydrates: White bread, pastries, cookies, and other meals containing refined flour may raise blood sugar levels and cause inflammation. Choose whole grain options that are high in fiber and nutrients.

3. Sugary Foods and Beverages: Added sugars, such as those found in soda, candy, and baked goods, may promote inflammation in the body. Limiting your consumption of these sweet delights might help keep inflammation under control.

4. Dairy products: For some people with vasculitis, dairy items such as milk, cheese, and yogurt might cause an immunological response and exacerbate inflammation. If you feel dairy is an issue for you, look into dairy-free alternatives.

5. Gluten-Containing Foods: Gluten, a protein present in wheat, rye, and barley, has been shown to aggravate inflammation in certain patients with autoimmune disorders such as vasculitis. Try a gluten-free diet to see if you feel better.

6. Nightshade Vegetables: The nightshade family includes tomatoes, potatoes, eggplants, and peppers, which might cause inflammation in certain vasculitis patients. If you discover that certain foods exacerbate your symptoms, it may be advisable to avoid them.

7. Alcohol: Excessive alcohol use might decrease immunological function and cause inflammation in the body. It's better to minimize or avoid drinking entirely, particularly during flare-ups.

Remember that everyone's body is unique, and what causes inflammation in one person may not affect another. It is important to pay careful attention to how your body reacts to various meals and make modifications appropriately.

Chapter 3

Quick and Healthy Anti-inflammatory Recipes

Breakfast Recipes

1. Acai Bowl with Granola and Coconut Flakes

• Total Time: 15 minutes • Serves: 3

Ingredients

- 1 cup frozen acai pulp
- 1 banana, sliced
- 1/2 cup unsweetened almond milk
- 1/4 cup granola (gluten-free, no added sugar)
- 2 tablespoons shredded unsweetened coconut

Procedure

1. In a high-speed blender, blend the frozen acai pulp, banana, and almond milk until smooth and creamy.
2. Divide the acai mixture evenly into 3 serving bowls.
3. Top each bowl with 2 tablespoons of granola and 2 teaspoons of shredded coconut.

Per serving: - Calories: 207 - Fiber: 7g - Carbs: 31g - Fats: 9g - Protein: 4g - Sugar: 15g

2. Blueberry Muffins with Almond Flour

• **Total Time: 35 minutes** • **Serves: 3**

Ingredients

- 1 1/2 cups almond flour
- 1/4 cup coconut flour
- 1 teaspoon baking powder
- 1/4 teaspoon baking soda
- 1/4 teaspoon sea salt
- 3 eggs
- 1/4 cup maple syrup
- 1/4 cup unsweetened almond milk
- 1 cup fresh or frozen blueberries

Procedure

1. Preheat your oven to 375°F (190°C). Grease a 9-cup muffin tin or line it with paper liners.
2. In a medium bowl, whisk together the almond flour, coconut flour, baking powder, baking soda, and salt.
3. In another bowl, beat the eggs, then stir in the maple syrup and almond milk.
4. Gently fold the wet ingredients into the dry ingredients until just combined. Fold in the blueberries.
5. Divide the batter evenly among the prepared muffin cups.
6. Bake for 18-20 minutes, or until a toothpick inserted in the center comes out clean.

Per serving: Calories:303 - Fiber: 6g - Carbs:25g - Fats: 19g - Protein: 11g - Sugar: 13g

3. Greek Yogurt Parfait with Granola

• **Total Time: 15 minutes • Serves: 3**

Ingredients

- 1 cup plain Greek yogurt
- 1/2 cup mixed berries (like blueberries, raspberries, and strawberries)
- 1/4 cup granola (gluten-free, no added sugar)

Procedure

1. In a serving glass or bowl, layer 1/3 cup of Greek yogurt, 2 tablespoons of mixed berries, and 1 tablespoon of granola.
2. Repeat the layers two more times to create 3 parfaits.

Per serving: Calories: 171 - Fiber: 3g - Carbs: 15g - Fats: 9g - Protein: 14g - Sugar: 11g

4. Mushroom and Spinach Frittata

• **Total Time: 40 minutes** • **Serves: 3**

Ingredients

- 6 eggs
- 1/4 cup unsweetened almond milk
- 1/4 teaspoon sea salt
- 1/8 teaspoon black pepper
- 1 tablespoon olive oil
- 8 ounces sliced mushrooms
- 2 cups fresh spinach
- 1/4 cup crumbled feta cheese (optional)

Procedure

1. Preheat your oven to 375°F (190°C).
2. In a medium bowl, whisk the eggs, almond milk, salt, and pepper.
3. Heat the olive oil in a 9-inch oven-safe skillet over medium heat. Add the mushrooms and sauté for 5-7 minutes until softened.
4. Add the spinach and sauté until wilted, about 2-3 minutes.
5. Pour the egg mixture over the mushrooms and spinach. Top with the feta cheese, if using.
6. Bake for 15-20 minutes, or until the frittata is set and lightly golden.

Per serving: Calories: 178 - Fiber: 2g - Carbs: 5g - Fats: 12g - Protein: 15g - Sugar: 2g

5. Oatmeal with Almond Butter and Bananas

• **Total Time: 30 minutes • Serves: 3**

Ingredients

- 1 cup rolled oats
- 2 cups unsweetened almond milk
- 2 tablespoons almond butter
- 1 banana, sliced
- 1 teaspoon cinnamon
- 1 tablespoon chia seeds (optional)

Procedure

1. In a medium saucepan, combine the rolled oats and almond milk. Bring to a simmer over medium heat, stirring occasionally.
2. Reduce the heat to low and continue cooking for 10-12 minutes, stirring occasionally, until the oats are tender and the mixture has thickened.
3. Remove from heat and stir in the almond butter until well combined.
4. Divide the oatmeal into 3 serving bowls. Top each with sliced banana, cinnamon, and chia seeds (optional).

Per serving: Calories: 280 - Fiber: 7g - Carbs: 37g - Fats: 13g - Protein: 9g - Sugar: 10g

6. Breakfast Salad with Poached Egg

• Total Time: 20 minutes • Serves: 3

Ingredients

- 6 cups mixed greens (spinach, arugula, kale)
- 3 eggs, poached
- 1 avocado, sliced
- 1/2 cup cherry tomatoes, halved
- 2 tbsp olive oil
- 1 tbsp apple cider vinegar
- Salt and pepper to taste

Procedure

1. Bring a pot of water to a gentle simmer. Crack the eggs into the simmering water and poach for 4-5 minutes until the whites are set but the yolks are still runny.
2. In a large bowl, combine the mixed greens, avocado slices, and cherry tomatoes.
3. Drizzle the olive oil and apple cider vinegar over the salad and toss gently to coat.
4. Season with salt and pepper.
5. Top each serving with a poached egg.

Per serving: Calories: 239 - Fiber: 7g - Carbs: 9g - Fats: 18g - Protein: 11g - Sugar: 2g

7. Breakfast Wrap with Turkey Bacon and Avocado

• **Total Time: 30 minutes** • **Serves: 3**

Ingredients

- 3 whole wheat tortillas
- 6 slices turkey bacon, cooked
- 1 avocado, mashed
- 3 tbsp plain Greek yogurt
- 1 cup baby spinach leaves
- Salt and pepper to taste

Procedure

1. Cook the turkey bacon according to package directions until crispy.
2. Warm the whole wheat tortillas.
3. Spread the mashed avocado evenly on each tortilla.
4. Top with 2 slices of turkey bacon, 1 tbsp of Greek yogurt, and a handful of baby spinach leaves.
5. Season with salt and pepper.
6. Fold the tortilla and enjoy.

Per serving: Calories:281 - Fiber: 6g - Carbs:27g - Fats: 16g - Protein: 17g - Sugar: 2g

8. Cottage Cheese with Fresh Berries

• **Total Time: 10 minutes** • **Serves: 3**

Ingredients

- 1 cup low-fat cottage cheese
- 1 cup mixed fresh berries (like blueberries, raspberries, strawberries)
- 1 tbsp honey (optional)

Procedure

1. Divide the cottage cheese evenly into three bowls.
2. Top each serving with a 1/3 cup of mixed fresh berries.
3. Drizzle 1 tsp of honey over the berries (optional).

Per serving: Calories: 123 - Fiber: 3g - Carbs: 12g - Fats: 5g - Protein: 14g - Sugar: 9g

9. Coconut Yogurt with Mixed Nuts and Seeds

• Total Time: 12 minutes • Serves: 3

Ingredients

- 1 1/2 cups unsweetened coconut yogurt
- 1/4 cup mixed nuts (like almonds, walnuts, cashews)
- 2 tbsp mixed seeds (like chia, flax, pumpkin)
- 1 tbsp honey (optional)

Procedure

1. Divide the coconut yogurt evenly into three bowls.
2. Top each serving with 1 tbsp of mixed nuts and 2 tsp of mixed seeds.
3. Drizzle 1 tsp of honey over the top (optional).

Per serving: Calories: 200 - Fiber: 4g - Carbs: 13g - Fats: 15g - Protein: 6g - Sugar: 7g

10. Whole Grain Pancakes with Maple Syrup

• Total Time: 30 minutes • Serves: 2

Ingredients

- 1 cup whole wheat flour
- 1 tsp baking powder
- 1/2 tsp baking soda
- 1/4 tsp salt
- 1 egg
- 1 cup unsweetened almond milk
- 1 tbsp pure maple syrup
- 1 tbsp avocado oil

Procedure

1. In a medium bowl, whisk together the whole wheat flour, baking powder, baking soda, and salt.
2. In another bowl, beat the egg, then stir in the almond milk, maple syrup, and avocado oil.
3. Pour the wet ingredients into the dry ingredients and stir just until combined (carefull, do not overmix).
4. Heat a nonstick skillet or griddle over medium heat. Scoop about 1/4 cup of batter per pancake onto the hot surface.
5. Cook for 2-3 minutes per side, or until golden brown.
6. Serve warm, drizzled with a little extra maple syrup if desired.

Per serving: Calories: 280 - Fiber: 5g - Carbs: 41g - Fats: 10g - Protein: 9g - Sugar: 12g

11. Sweet Potato Hash with Eggs

• Total Time: 40 minutes • Serves: 3

Ingredients

- 2 medium sweet potatoes, diced
- 1 tablespoon olive oil
- 1 small onion, diced
- 2 cloves garlic, minced
- 1 teaspoon ground cumin
- 1/2 teaspoon smoked paprika
- Salt and pepper to taste
- 6 eggs

Procedure

1. In a large skillet, heat the olive oil over medium heat.
2. Add the diced sweet potatoes, onion, garlic, cumin, and smoked paprika. Season with salt and pepper.
3. Cook, (stirring occasionally) for 15-20 minutes until the sweet potatoes are tender.
4. Create 6 wells in the hash and crack the eggs into them.
5. Cover the skillet and cook for 5-7 minutes until the eggs are set.
6. Serve immediately and enjoy.

Per serving: Calories:298 - Fiber: 5g - Carbs:30g - Fats: 14g - Protein: 16g - Sugar: 7g

12. Green Smoothie with Kale and Pineapple

• **Total Time: 10 minutes** • **Serves: 3**

Ingredients

- 2 cups packed kale leaves
- 1 cup frozen pineapple chunks
- 1 banana
- 1 cup unsweetened almond milk
- 1 tablespoon honey (optional)

Procedure

1. Add all ingredients to your high-speed blender.
2. Blend on high speed until smooth and creamy.
3. Pour into glasses and enjoy immediately.

Per serving: - Calories: 151 - Fiber: 4g - Carbs: 33g - Fats: 2g - Protein: 3g
- Sugar: 20g

13. Buckwheat Porridge with Cinnamon and Apples

• Total Time: 30 minutes • Serves: 3

Ingredients

- 1 cup raw buckwheat groats
- 2 cups unsweetened almond milk
- 1 teaspoon ground cinnamon
- 1 medium apple, diced
- 2 tablespoons raw honey (optional)

Procedure

1. In a medium saucepan, combine the buckwheat groats and almond milk. Bring to a boil.
2. Reduce heat to low, cover and simmer for 15-20 minutes, stirring occasionally, until the buckwheat is tender and the porridge thickens.
3. Remove from heat and stir in the cinnamon, diced apple, and honey (optional).
4. Serve warm and enjoy!

Per serving: - Calories: 223 - Fiber: 5g - Carbs: 39g - Fats: 6g - Protein: 6g - Sugar: 15g

14. Peanut Butter Banana Protein Shake

• Total Time: 10 minutes • Serves: 3

Ingredients

- 2 ripe bananas
- 1/2 cup creamy peanut butter
- 1 cup unsweetened almond milk
- 1 scoop vanilla protein powder
- 1 tablespoon ground flaxseed

Procedure

1. Add all ingredients to your high-speed blender.
2. Blend on high speed until smooth and creamy.
3. Pour into glasses and serve immediately.

Per serving: Calories:315 - Fiber: 6g - Carbs:29g - Fats: 18g - Protein: 16g - Sugar: 12g

15. Breakfast Tacos with Avocado and Salsa

• Total Time: 20 minutes • Serves: 3

Ingredients

- 6 small corn tortillas
- 6 eggs, scrambled
- 1 avocado, sliced
- 1/2 cup pico de gallo (or salsa)
- 1 tablespoon chopped cilantro

Procedure

1. Warm the corn tortillas according to package directions.
2. In a skillet, scramble the eggs until cooked through.
3. To assemble, place the scrambled eggs in the center of each tortilla.
4. Top with sliced avocado, pico de gallo/salsa, and chopped cilantro.
5. Serve immediately and enjoy!

Per serving: Calories:271 - Fiber: 7g - Carbs:25g - Fats: 15g - Protein: 14g - Sugar: 2g

Lunch Recipes

---

1. Greek Orzo Salad with Feta

• **Total Time: 50 minutes** • **Serves: 5**

Ingredients

- 1 cup uncooked orzo pasta
- 1 cup cherry tomatoes, halved
- 1 cucumber, diced
- 1/2 cup crumbled feta cheese
- 1/4 cup sliced black olives
- 2 tablespoons fresh parsley, chopped
- 2 tablespoons fresh lemon juice
- 1 tablespoon olive oil
- 1 teaspoon dried oregano
- Salt and pepper to taste

Procedure

1. Cook the orzo according to package directions. Drain and rinse with cold water.
2. In a large bowl, combine the cooked orzo, cherry tomatoes, cucumber, feta cheese, black olives, and parsley.
3. In a small bowl, whisk together the lemon juice, olive oil, oregano, salt, and pepper.
4. Pour the dressing over the salad and toss gently to coat.
5. Serve chilled or at room temperature.

Per serving: - Calories: 180 - Fiber: 3g - Carbs: 25g - Fats: 8g - Protein: 6g - Sugar: 3g

2. Lentil Soup with Spinach

• **Total Time: 50 minutes • Serves: 5**

Ingredients

- 1 tablespoon olive oil
- 1 onion, diced
- 3 garlic cloves, minced
- 1 cup brown lentils, rinsed
- 4 cups low-sodium vegetable broth
- 1 (14.5 oz) can diced tomatoes
- 1 teaspoon dried thyme
- 1 teaspoon dried basil
- Salt and pepper to taste
- 2 cups fresh spinach, chopped

Procedure

1. In a large pot, heat the olive oil over medium heat. Add the onion and sauté for 5 minutes until translucent.
2. Add the garlic and sauté for another minute until fragrant.
3. Stir in the lentils, vegetable broth, diced tomatoes, thyme, and basil. Bring to a boil.
4. Reduce heat and simmer for 20-25 minutes, or until the lentils are tender.
5. Stir in the chopped spinach and cook for an additional 2-3 minutes until the spinach is wilted.
6. Season with salt and pepper to taste.
7. Serve hot and enjoy!

Per serving: Calories:220 - Fiber: 10g - Carbs:33g - Fats: 5g - Protein: 13g - Sugar: 6g

3. Baked Salmon with Roasted Vegetables

• Total Time: 45 minutes • Serves: 5

Ingredients

- 1 lb salmon fillets (cut into 5 portions)
- 2 cups broccoli florets
- 2 cups cauliflower florets
- 1 red bell pepper, sliced
- 1 zucchini, sliced
- 2 tablespoons olive oil
- 1 teaspoon garlic powder
- 1 teaspoon dried dill
- Salt and pepper to taste

Procedure

1. Preheat your oven to 400°F.
2. Arrange the salmon fillets and the vegetables on a large baking sheet. Drizzle with olive oil and sprinkle with garlic powder, dried dill, salt, and pepper.
3. Bake for 20-25 minutes, or until the salmon is cooked through and the vegetables are tender.
4. Serve the baked salmon with the roasted vegetables.

Per serving: Calories:300 - Fiber: 5g - Carbs:10g - Fats: 18g - Protein: 30g - Sugar: 4g

4. Chickpea Salad with Lemon Dressing

• **Total Time: 30 minutes** • **Serves: 5**

Ingredients

- 2 (15 oz) cans chickpeas (rinsed and drained)
- 1 cup diced cucumber
- 1/2 cup diced red onion
- 1/4 cup chopped fresh parsley
- 2 tablespoons lemon juice
- 1 tablespoon olive oil
- 1 teaspoon Dijon mustard
- Salt and pepper to taste

Procedure

1. In a large bowl, combine the chickpeas, cucumber, red onion, and parsley.
2. In a small bowl, whisk together the lemon juice, olive oil, and Dijon mustard.
3. Pour the dressing over the chickpea salad and toss gently to coat.
4. Season with salt and pepper to taste.
5. Serve chilled or at room temperature.

Per serving: - Calories: 180 - Fiber: 6g - Carbs: 26g - Fats: 6g - Protein: 8g - Sugar: 3g

5. Broccoli and Cheddar Soup

• Total Time: 30 minutes • Serves: 5

Ingredients

- 2 tablespoons olive oil
- 1 onion, diced
- 2 garlic cloves, minced
- 4 cups low-sodium vegetable broth
- 3 cups broccoli florets
- 1 cup shredded cheddar cheese
- 1/4 cup unsweetened almond milk
- 1 tablespoon cornstarch
- Salt and pepper to taste

Procedure

1. In a large pot, heat the olive oil over medium heat. Add the onion and sauté for 5 minutes until translucent.
2. Add the garlic and sauté for another minute until fragrant.
3. Pour in the vegetable broth and add the broccoli florets. Bring to a boil, then reduce heat and simmer for 10-15 minutes, or until the broccoli is tender.
4. In a small bowl, whisk together the almond milk and cornstarch.
5. Carefully take the soup to a blender and blend until smooth. Return the blended soup to the pot.
6. Stir in the almond milk mixture and the shredded cheddar cheese. Cook for 2-3 minutes, or until the cheese is melted and the soup has thickened.
7. Season with salt and pepper to taste. Serve hot and enjoy!

Per serving: Calories:190 - Fiber: 4g - Carbs:13g - Fats: 12g - Protein: 11g - Sugar: 3g

6. Falafel Salad with Tahini Dressing

• Total Time: 50 minutes • Serves: 4

Ingredients

Falafel:
- 1 (15 oz) can chickpeas (drained and rinsed)
- 1/2 cup fresh parsley, chopped
- 2 cloves garlic, minced
- 1 tsp ground cumin
- 1/2 tsp ground coriander
- 1/4 tsp cayenne pepper
- 1/4 cup whole wheat breadcrumbs
- 1 tbsp olive oil

Salad:
- 5 cups mixed greens
- 1 cup cherry tomatoes, halved
- 1/2 cucumber, sliced
- 1/4 red onion (thinly sliced)

Tahini Dressing:
- 1/4 cup tahini
- 2 tbsp lemon juice
- 2 tbsp water
- 1 tbsp maple syrup
- 1 clove garlic, minced
- 1/4 tsp salt

Procedure

1. Preheat your oven to 400°F. Line a baking sheet with parchment paper.

Falafel:
1. In a food processor, combine the chickpeas, parsley, garlic, cumin, coriander, and cayenne. Pulse until coarsely chopped.
2. Take the mixture to a bowl and stir in the breadcrumbs.
3. Form the mixture into 12 small patties, about 2 tbsp each.
4. Heat the olive oil in a large non-stick skillet over medium heat. Add the falafel patties and cook for 2-3 minutes per side until golden brown.
5. Take the cooked falafel to the prepared baking sheet and bake for 10 minutes.

Salad:
1. In a large bowl, combine the mixed greens, cherry tomatoes, cucumber, and red onion.

Tahini Dressing:
1. In a small bowl, whisk together the tahini, lemon juice, water, maple syrup, garlic, and salt until smooth.

Assembly:
1. Divide the salad greens among 4 plates.
2. Top each salad with 3 falafel patties.
3. Drizzle the tahini dressing over the top.

Per serving: Calories: 334 - Fiber: 8g - Carbs: 39g - Fat: 16g - Protein: 13g - Sugar: 9g

7. Tuna Salad Lettuce Wraps

• Total Time: 20 minutes • Serves: 5

Ingredients

- 2 (5 oz) cans of tuna, drained
- 1/4 cup plain Greek yogurt
- 1 tbsp Dijon mustard
- 1 tbsp lemon juice
- 2 tbsp chopped green onions
- 1/4 cup diced celery
- 1/4 tsp salt
- 1/4 tsp black pepper
- 10 large lettuce leaves (like romaine or bibb)

Procedure

1. In a medium bowl, mix together the tuna, Greek yogurt, Dijon mustard, lemon juice, green onions, celery, salt, and pepper until well combined.
2. Spoon the tuna salad mixture evenly into the lettuce leaves.
3. Serve immediately and enjoy!

Per serving: - Calories: 117 - Fiber: 2g - Carbs: 4g - Fats: 4g - Protein: 16g - Sugar: 2g

8. Black Bean and Corn Quesadillas

• Total Time: 30 minutes • Serves: 5

Ingredients

- 1 (15 oz) can black beans (rinsed and drained)
- 1 cup frozen corn, thawed
- 1/4 cup diced red onion
- 1 tbsp lime juice
- 1 tsp ground cumin
- 1/4 tsp salt
- 10 whole-wheat tortillas
- 1 cup shredded cheddar cheese

Procedure

1. In a medium bowl, add the black beans, corn, red onion, lime juice, cumin, and salt. Stir to mix well.
2. Place a tortilla on a flat surface. Spread about 1/2 cup of the black bean and corn mixture evenly over half of the tortilla. Sprinkle with 2 tbsp of shredded cheddar cheese.
3. Fold the other half of the tortilla over the filling to create a half-moon shape.
4. Heat a large skillet or griddle over medium heat. Cook the quesadillas in batches for 2-3 minutes per side, or until the tortilla is golden brown and the cheese is melted.
5. Cut the quesadillas in half and serve immediately.

Per serving: Calories:320 - Fiber: 8g - Carbs:42g - Fats: 11g - Protein: 15g - Sugar: 2g

9. Mediterranean Pasta Salad

• Total Time: 50 minutes • Serves: 5

Ingredients

- 8 oz whole-wheat pasta (cooked according to package directions)
- 1 cup cherry tomatoes, halved
- 1 cucumber, diced
- 1/2 cup pitted kalamata olives, sliced
- 1/4 cup crumbled feta cheese
- 2 tbsp chopped fresh parsley
- 2 tbsp olive oil
- 2 tbsp red wine vinegar
- 1 tsp Dijon mustard
- 1 tsp dried oregano
- 1/4 tsp salt
- 1/4 tsp black pepper

Procedure

1. In a large bowl, combine the cooked and cooled pasta, cherry tomatoes, cucumber, olives, feta cheese, and parsley.
2. In a small bowl, whisk together the olive oil, red wine vinegar, Dijon mustard, oregano, salt, and pepper.
3. Pour the dressing over the pasta salad and toss gently to coat.
4. Refrigerate for at least 30 minutes to allow the flavors to meld.
5. Serve chilled or at room temperature.

Per serving: Calories: 262 - Fiber: 5g - Carbs: 34g - Fats: 11g - Protein: 8g - Sugar: 3g

10. BBQ Chicken and Pineapple Skewers

• Total Time: 35 minutes • Serves: 4

Ingredients

- 1 lb boneless, skinless chicken breasts (cut into 1-inch cubes)
- 1 cup fresh pineapple chunks
- 1 red bell pepper (cut into 1-inch pieces)
- 1 yellow onion (cut into 1-inch pieces)
- 2 tbsp olive oil
- 1/4 cup low-sodium barbecue sauce
- Salt and black pepper to taste

Procedure

1. Preheat a grill or grill pan to medium-high heat.
2. In a large bowl, toss the chicken, pineapple, bell pepper, and onion with the olive oil. Season with salt and pepper.
3. Thread the chicken and vegetables onto skewers, alternating the ingredients.
4. Grill the skewers for 12-15 minutes, turning occasionally, until the chicken is cooked through.
5. Brush the skewers with the barbecue sauce during the last 2-3 minutes of cooking.
6. Serve immediately and enjoy!

Per serving: - Calories: 258 - Fiber: 2g - Carbs: 17g - Fat: 9g - Protein: 28g - Sugar: 12g

11. Zucchini Noodles with Pesto and Cherry Tomatoes

• **Total Time: 20 minutes** • **Serves: 3**

Ingredients

- 3 medium zucchinis (spiralized or julienned)
- 1 cup cherry tomatoes, halved
- 1/2 cup homemade basil pesto
- 2 tbsp pine nuts
- 1/4 cup grated Parmesan cheese (optional)
- Salt and pepper to taste

Procedure

1. In a large bowl, combine the spiralized zucchini noodles and cherry tomatoes.
2. Add the basil pesto and toss to coat the noodles evenly.
3. Top with pine nuts and Parmesan cheese (optional).
4. Season with salt and pepper to taste.

Per serving: - Calories: 167 - Fiber: 3.5g - Carbs: 8.5g - Fats: 13.5g - Protein: 6.7g - Sugar: 4.5g

12. Salmon and Asparagus Foil Packets

• Total Time: 35 minutes • Serves: 3

Ingredients

- 3 salmon fillets (4-6 oz each)
- 1 lb asparagus, trimmed
- 2 tbsp olive oil
- 2 tbsp lemon juice
- 1 tsp garlic powder
- 1 tsp dried dill
- Salt and pepper to taste

Procedure

1. Preheat your oven to 400°F.
2. Cut 3 large sheets of foil and place an equal amount of asparagus in the center of each sheet.
3. Top the asparagus with a salmon fillet.
4. Drizzle with olive oil and lemon juice, and season with garlic powder, dried dill, salt, and pepper.
5. Fold the foil over the salmon and asparagus and seal the edges to create a tight packet.
6. Bake for 18-20 minutes, or until the salmon is cooked through and the asparagus is tender.

Per serving: Calories:261 - Fiber: 3.5g - Carbs:4g - Fats:15g - Protein: 28g - Sugar: 1g

13. Lemon Herb Chicken Salad

• Total Time: 30 minutes • Serves: 3

Ingredients

- 2 cups cooked and shredded chicken breast
- 1/4 cup plain Greek yogurt
- 2 tbsp lemon juice
- 1 tbsp Dijon mustard
- 1 tsp dried parsley
- 1 tsp dried dill
- 1/4 cup diced celery
- 2 tbsp chopped green onions
- Salt and pepper to taste

Procedure

1. In a large bowl, add the shredded chicken, Greek yogurt, lemon juice, Dijon mustard, dried parsley, and dried dill.
2. Gently mix until the chicken is evenly coated.
3. Fold in the diced celery and chopped green onions.
4. Season with salt and pepper to taste.
5. Serve on a bed of greens or in lettuce wraps.

Per serving: - Calories: 182 - Fiber: 1g - Carbs: 3g - Fats: 7g - Protein: 26g - Sugar: 2g

14. Eggplant Parmesan with Whole Wheat Pasta

• Total Time: 60 minutes • Serves: 3

Ingredients

- 1 medium eggplant (sliced into 1/2-inch rounds)
- 1 cup marinara sauce
- 1/2 cup shredded mozzarella cheese
- 1/4 cup grated Parmesan cheese
- 2 tbsp olive oil
- 1 tsp dried oregano
- 1/2 tsp garlic powder
- Salt and pepper to taste
- 8 oz whole wheat pasta (cooked according to package directions)

Procedure

1. Preheat your oven to 400°F.
2. Arrange the eggplant slices on a baking sheet and brush both sides with olive oil. Season with salt, pepper, and garlic powder.
3. Bake for 20-25 minutes, flipping halfway, until the eggplant is tender and lightly browned.
4. In a baking dish, layer the baked eggplant slices, then top with marinara sauce, mozzarella, and Parmesan cheese.
5. Bake for an additional 15-20 minutes, or until the cheese is melted and bubbly.
6. Serve the eggplant Parmesan over the cooked whole wheat pasta.

Per serving: Calories:346 - Fiber:10g - Carbs:41g - Fats:15g - Protein: 19g - Sugar: 8g

15. Cauliflower Crust Pizza with Arugula and Prosciutto

• Total Time: 60 minutes • Serves: 3

Ingredients

Cauliflower Crust:
- 3 cups riced cauliflower (about 1 medium head)
- 1 egg, beaten
- 1/4 cup grated Parmesan cheese
- 1/4 tsp garlic powder
- 1/4 tsp dried oregano
- Salt and pepper to taste

Toppings:
- 1/2 cup marinara sauce
- 1 cup shredded mozzarella cheese
- 3 oz prosciutto (thinly sliced)
- 2 cups arugula

Procedure

1. Preheat your oven to 400°F. Line a baking sheet with parchment paper.
2. Make the cauliflower crust: In a food processor, pulse the cauliflower florets until they resemble rice. Transfer to a clean kitchen towel and squeeze out as much moisture as possible.
3. In a bowl, mix the riced cauliflower, beaten egg, Parmesan, garlic powder, oregano, salt, and pepper until well combined.
4. Press the cauliflower mixture onto the prepared baking sheet, forming a thin, even crust.
5. Bake for 20-25 minutes, or until the crust is golden brown.

6. Remove the crust from the oven and top with the marinara sauce, mozzarella cheese, and prosciutto.
7. Bake for an additional 10-12 minutes, or until the cheese is melted and bubbly.
8. Top the pizza with the arugula and serve.

Per serving: Calories:276 - Fiber: 4g - Carbs:16g - Fats: 16g - Protein: 21g - Sugar: 6g

Dinner Recipes

1. Blackened Mahi Mahi with Mango Salsa

• **Total Time: 40 minutes • Serves: 5**

Ingredients

- 5 (6 oz) mahi mahi fillets
- 2 tbsp blackened seasoning
- 1 mango, diced
- 1 red bell pepper, diced
- 1/2 cup diced red onion
- 1 jalapeño, seeded and diced
- 2 tbsp freshly chopped cilantro
- 2 tbsp lime juice
- 1 tsp olive oil

Procedure

1. Preheat your oven to 400°F.
2. Season the mahi mahi fillets evenly with the blackened seasoning.
3. Place the seasoned fillets on a baking sheet lined with parchment paper.
4. Bake for 15-18 minutes, or until the fish flakes easily with a fork.
5. In a medium bowl, add the diced mango, bell pepper, red onion, jalapeño, cilantro, lime juice, and olive oil. Mix well.
6. Serve the blackened mahi mahi with the fresh mango salsa.

Per serving: Calories: 250 - Fiber: 3g - Carbs: 15g - Fats: 9g - Protein: 30g - Sugar: 9g

2. Baked Chicken and Vegetable Stir-Fry

• **Total Time: 50 minutes** • **Serves: 5**

Ingredients

- 5 (6 oz) boneless, skinless chicken breasts (cubed)
- 2 cups broccoli florets
- 1 cup sliced mushrooms
- 1 red bell pepper, sliced
- 1 cup snow peas
- 2 tbsp low-sodium soy sauce
- 1 tbsp sesame oil
- 2 tsp minced garlic
- 1 tsp grated fresh ginger
- 1/4 tsp red pepper flakes (optional)

Procedure

1. Preheat your oven to 400°F.
2. In a large bowl, combine the cubed chicken, broccoli, mushrooms, bell pepper, and snow peas.
3. In a small bowl, whisk together the soy sauce, sesame oil, garlic, ginger, and red pepper flakes (optional).
4. Pour the sauce over the chicken and vegetables and toss to coat.
5. Spread the mixture on a baking sheet lined with parchment paper.
6. Bake for 25-30 minutes, or until the chicken is cooked through and the vegetables are tender.

Per serving: Calories: 220 - Fiber: 4g - Carbs: 11g - Fats: 7g - Protein: 28g - Sugar: 4g

3. Hawaiian Chicken Pineapple Bowls

• Total Time: 50 minutes • Serves: 5

Ingredients

- 5 (6 oz) boneless, skinless chicken breasts (cubed)
- 1 cup diced pineapple
- 1 red bell pepper, diced
- 1 cup diced red onion
- 2 tbsp low-sodium soy sauce
- 1 tbsp rice vinegar
- 1 tsp sesame oil
- 1 tsp grated fresh ginger
- 1/4 tsp red pepper flakes (optional)
- 5 small pineapple halves (for serving)

Procedure

1. Preheat your oven to 400°F.
2. In a large bowl, combine the cubed chicken, diced pineapple, bell pepper, and red onion.
3. In a small bowl, whisk together the soy sauce, rice vinegar, sesame oil, ginger, and red pepper flakes (optional).
4. Pour the sauce over the chicken and vegetable mixture and toss to coat.
5. Spread the mixture on a baking sheet lined with parchment paper.
6. Bake for 25-30 minutes, or until the chicken is cooked through.
7. Serve the baked chicken and vegetable mixture in the pineapple halves.

Per serving: Calories: 280 - Fiber: 3g - Carbs: 20g - Fats: 8g - Protein: 30g - Sugar: 14g

4. Baked Chicken with Sweet Potato Mash

• **Total Time: 60 minutes • Serves: 5**

Ingredients

- 5 (6 oz) boneless, skinless chicken breasts
- 3 medium sweet potatoes (peeled and cubed)
- 2 tbsp olive oil, divided
- 1 tsp garlic powder
- 1 tsp paprika
- 1/2 tsp dried thyme
- Salt and black pepper (to taste)
- 1/4 cup unsweetened almond milk
- 2 tbsp chopped fresh parsley

Procedure

1. Preheat your oven to 400°F.
2. Place the chicken breasts on a baking sheet lined with parchment paper.
3. In a large bowl, toss the cubed sweet potatoes with 1 tbsp of olive oil, garlic powder, paprika, dried thyme, salt, and black pepper.
4. Spread the seasoned sweet potatoes on a separate baking sheet.
5. Bake the chicken and sweet potatoes for 25-30 minutes, or until the chicken is cooked through and the sweet potatoes are tender.
6. In a medium saucepan, mash the cooked sweet potatoes with the remaining 1 tbsp of olive oil and the almond milk until smooth.
7. Serve the baked chicken with the sweet potato mash, garnished with fresh parsley.

Per serving: Calories:320 - Fiber: 5g - Carbs:25g - Fats: 10g - Protein: 35g - Sugar: 7g

5. Seared Tuna with Cucumber Salad

• Total Time: 30 minutes • Serves: 5

Ingredients

- 5 (6 oz) tuna steaks
- 2 tbsp olive oil
- 1 tsp sesame seeds
- 1 tsp black pepper
- 1 cucumber, sliced
- 1/2 red onion, thinly sliced
- 2 tbsp rice vinegar
- 1 tbsp sesame oil
- 1 tbsp grated fresh ginger
- 1 tbsp chopped fresh cilantro

Procedure

1. Season the tuna steaks with sesame seeds and black pepper.
2. Heat 1 tbsp of olive oil in a large skillet over high heat.
3. Sear the tuna steaks for 2-3 minutes per side, or until the outside is lightly charred but the center is still rare. Transfer to a plate.
4. In a medium bowl, combine the sliced cucumber, red onion, rice vinegar, 1 tbsp sesame oil, grated ginger, and chopped cilantro. Toss to coat.
5. Slice the seared tuna steaks and serve with the cucumber salad.

Per serving: Calories: 260 - Fiber: 2g - Carbs: 6g - Fats: 14g - Protein: 28g - Sugar: 3g

6. Roasted Garlic Cauliflower Soup

• **Total Time: 60 minutes • Serves: 5**

Ingredients

- 1 head of cauliflower, cut into florets (about 4 cups)
- 4 cloves of garlic, minced   - 1 onion, diced
- 4 cups of low-sodium vegetable (or chicken broth)
- 1 cup of unsweetened almond milk   - 2 tbsp of extra virgin olive oil
- 1 tsp of dried thyme   - Salt and pepper to taste

Procedure

1. Preheat your oven to 400°F (200°C).
2. Spread the cauliflower florets and minced garlic on a baking sheet. Drizzle with 1 tbsp of olive oil and season with salt and pepper.
3. Roast for 20-25 minutes, or until the cauliflower is tender and lightly browned.
4. In a large saucepan, heat the remaining 1 tbsp of olive oil over medium heat. Add the diced onion and sauté for 5-7 minutes, until translucent.
5. Add the roasted cauliflower and garlic to the saucepan. Pour in the vegetable or chicken broth and stir in the dried thyme.
6. Bring the mixture to a boil, then reduce the heat and let it simmer for 10-15 minutes.
7. Carefully take the soup to a blender or use an immersion blender to puree the soup until smooth.
8. Stir in the unsweetened almond milk and adjust the seasoning with salt and pepper to taste.

Per serving: - Calories: 125 - Fiber: 4g - Carbs: 13g - Fats: 7g - Protein: 4g - Sugar: 4g

7. Lemon Herb Roasted Chicken Thighs

• Total Time: 60 minutes • Serves: 5

Ingredients

- 10 chicken thighs (bone-in, skin-on)
- 2 tbsp of lemon juice
- 2 tbsp of fresh chopped parsley
- 2 tbsp of fresh chopped rosemary
- 2 tbsp of extra virgin olive oil
- 1 tsp of garlic powder
- Salt and pepper to taste

Procedure

1. Preheat your oven to 400°F (200°C).
2. In a large bowl, add the lemon juice, parsley, rosemary, olive oil, garlic powder, salt, and pepper. Mix well.
3. Add the chicken thighs to the bowl and toss to coat them evenly with the herb mixture.
4. Arrange the chicken thighs on a baking sheet lined with parchment paper.
5. Roast the chicken for 35-40 minutes, or until the internal temperature reaches 165°F (75°C).
6. Serve the lemon herb roasted chicken thighs hot.

Per serving: Calories: 291 - Fiber: 0g - Carbs: 1g - Fats: 19g - Protein: 33g - Sugar: 0g

8. Spaghetti Squash with Turkey Bolognese

• **Total Time: 1 hour 15 minutes • Serves: 5**

Ingredients

- 1 medium spaghetti squash (halved and seeded)
- 1 lb of ground turkey
- 1 onion, diced
- 3 cloves of garlic, minced
- 1 can (28 oz) of crushed tomatoes
- 2 tbsp of tomato paste
- 1 tsp of dried oregano
- 1 tsp of dried basil
- Salt and pepper to taste

Procedure

1. Preheat your oven to 400°F (200°C).
2. Place the spaghetti squash halves cut-side down on a baking sheet. Roast for 40-45 minutes, or until the squash is tender and can be easily shredded with a fork.
3. In a large skillet, cook the ground turkey over medium heat, breaking it up with a wooden spoon, until no longer pink, about 5-7 minutes.
4. Add the diced onion and minced garlic to the skillet and sauté for 3-4 minutes, until the onion is translucent.
5. Stir in the crushed tomatoes, tomato paste, dried oregano, and dried basil. Season with salt and pepper to taste.
6. Reduce the heat and let the bolognese simmer for 15-20 minutes, stirring occasionally, until the flavors have melded.
7. Use a fork to shred the roasted spaghetti squash and divide it among plates.
8. Top the spaghetti squash with the turkey bolognese sauce and serve.

Per serving: Calories: 235 - Fiber: 5g - Carbs: 23g - Fats: 9g - Protein: 21g - Sugar: 8g

9. Ginger Soy Glazed Cod

• **Total Time: 35 minutes** • **Serves: 5**

Ingredients

- 5 (6 oz) cod fillets
- 2 tbsp of low-sodium soy sauce
- 2 tbsp of honey
- 1 tbsp of freshly grated ginger
- 1 tbsp of rice vinegar
- 1 tsp of sesame oil
- Salt and pepper to taste
- 2 tbsp of chopped green onions (for garnish)

Procedure

1. Preheat your oven to 400°F (200°C).
2. In a small bowl, whisk together the soy sauce, honey, grated ginger, rice vinegar, and sesame oil.
3. Place the cod fillets in a baking dish and season with salt and pepper.
4. Spoon the ginger-soy glaze over the cod, making sure to coat the fish evenly.
5. Bake the cod for 15-20 minutes, or until the fish flakes easily with a fork.
6. Garnish the ginger soy glazed cod with chopped green onions before serving.

Per serving: Calories: 195 - Fiber: 0g - Carbs: 10g - Fats: 4g - Protein: 27g - Sugar: 8g

10. Greek Chicken Souvlaki Skewers

• Total Time: 60 minutes • Serves: 5

Ingredients

- 1 lb of boneless, skinless chicken breasts (cut into 1-inch cubes)
- 2 tbsp of lemon juice
- 2 tbsp of extra virgin olive oil
- 1 tbsp of dried oregano
- 2 cloves of garlic, minced
- Salt and pepper to taste
- 1 red onion (cut into 1-inch pieces)
- 1 red bell pepper (cut into 1-inch pieces)
- 1 yellow bell pepper (cut into 1-inch pieces)

Procedure

1. In a large bowl, add the cubed chicken, lemon juice, olive oil, dried oregano, minced garlic, salt, and pepper. Mix well and let the chicken marinate for 30 minutes.
2. Preheat a grill or oven to 400°F (200°C).
3. Thread the marinated chicken cubes, red onion pieces, and bell pepper pieces onto skewers, alternating the ingredients.
4. Grill the skewers for 12-15 minutes, turning occasionally, or until the chicken is cooked through and the vegetables are tender.
5. Serve the Greek chicken souvlaki skewers hot.

Per serving: - Calories: 210 - Fiber: 2g - Carbs: 8g - Fats: 8g - Protein: 26g - Sugar: 4g

11. Mushroom and Spinach Quinoa Risotto

• **Total Time: 45 minutes** • **Serves: 3**

Ingredients

- 1 cup uncooked quinoa, rinsed
- 3 cups low-sodium vegetable broth
- 8 oz sliced mushrooms
- 2 cups fresh spinach, chopped
- 2 cloves garlic, minced
- 1 tbsp olive oil
- 2 tbsp grated Parmesan cheese (optional)
- Salt and pepper to taste

Procedure

1. In a medium saucepan, combine the quinoa and vegetable broth. Bring to a boil, then reduce heat and simmer for 15-20 minutes, or until quinoa is tender and liquid is absorbed.
2. In a large skillet, heat the olive oil over medium heat. Add the sliced mushrooms and sauté for 5-7 minutes, until they start to brown.
3. Add the minced garlic and sauté for an additional minute.
4. Add the cooked quinoa and chopped spinach to the skillet. Stir until the spinach is wilted, about 2-3 minutes.
5. Season with salt and pepper to taste.
6. Serve warm, and top with Parmesan cheese (optional).

Per serving: Calories: 239 - Fiber: 5g - Carbs: 36g - Fats: 7g - Protein: 10g - Sugar: 2g

12. Baked Cod with Tomato and Olive Relish

• Total Time: 35 minutes • Serves: 3

Ingredients

- 1 lb cod fillets
- 1 cup diced tomatoes
- 1/4 cup pitted and sliced black olives
- 2 tbsp chopped fresh parsley
- 1 tbsp olive oil
- 1 tbsp lemon juice
- Salt and pepper to taste

Procedure

1. Preheat your oven to 400°F.
2. Place the cod fillets in a baking dish and season with salt and pepper.
3. In a small bowl, combine the diced tomatoes, sliced black olives, chopped parsley, olive oil, and lemon juice. Mix well.
4. Spoon the tomato and olive relish over the cod fillets.
5. Bake for 15-20 minutes, or until the cod is cooked through and flakes easily with a fork.
6. Serve the baked cod with the tomato and olive relish.

Per serving: - Calories: 175 - Fiber: 2g - Carbs: 5g - Fats: 7g - Protein: 24g - Sugar: 2g

13. Butternut Squash and Black Bean Enchiladas

• **Total Time: 60 minutes** • **Serves: 3**

Ingredients

- 1 small butternut squash (peeled and diced)
- 1 can (15 oz) black beans (rinsed and drained)
- 1 cup shredded Mexican-blend cheese (optional)
- 8 small whole wheat tortillas
- 1 jar (16 oz) low-sodium enchilada sauce
- 1 tsp ground cumin
- Salt and pepper to taste

Procedure

1. Preheat your oven to 375°F.
2. In a medium saucepan, steam the diced butternut squash until tender, about 10 minutes. Drain and mash lightly.
3. In a bowl, combine the mashed butternut squash, black beans, and cumin. Season with salt and pepper.
4. Spread a thin layer of enchilada sauce in the bottom of a 9x13 inch baking dish.
5. Spoon the butternut squash and black bean mixture into the center of each tortilla. Roll up the tortillas and place seam-side down in the baking dish.
6. Pour the remaining enchilada sauce over the top of the rolled enchiladas.
7. Sprinkle the shredded cheese over the top, if using.
8. Bake for 20-25 minutes, or until heated through and the cheese is melted. Serve hot and enjoy!

Per serving: Calories:342 - Fiber: 10g - Carbs:51g - Fats: 8g - Protein: 15g - Sugar: 5g

14. Lemon Dill Shrimp and Asparagus Stir-Fry

• Total Time: 30 minutes • Serves: 3

Ingredients

- 1 lb shrimp, peeled and deveined
- 1 lb asparagus (trimmed and cut into 1-inch pieces)
- 2 tbsp olive oil
- 2 cloves garlic, minced
- 1 tbsp lemon juice
- 2 tsp chopped fresh dill
- Salt and pepper to taste

Procedure

1. In a large skillet or wok, heat the olive oil over medium-high heat.
2. Add the shrimp and asparagus to the skillet. Sauté for 5-7 minutes, stirring occasionally, until the shrimp are opaque and the asparagus is tender-crisp.
3. Add the minced garlic and sauté for an additional minute.
4. Stir in the lemon juice and chopped fresh dill. Season with salt and pepper to taste.
5. Serve immediately and enjoy!

Per serving: - Calories: 190 - Fiber: 3g - Carbs: 6g - Fats: 8g - Protein: 23g - Sugar: 2g

15. Sweet Potato and Black Bean Chili

• **Total Time: 50 minutes** • **Serves: 3**

Ingredients

- 1 lb sweet potatoes (peeled and diced)
- 1 can (15 oz) black beans (rinsed and drained)
- 1 can (15 oz) diced tomatoes
- 1 cup low-sodium vegetable broth
- 1 tbsp chili powder
- 1 tsp ground cumin
- 1 tsp smoked paprika
- 1/2 tsp garlic powder
- Salt and pepper to taste
- Chopped cilantro for garnish (optional)

Procedure

1. In a large pot or Dutch oven, combine the diced sweet potatoes, black beans, diced tomatoes, and vegetable broth.
2. Add the chili powder, cumin, smoked paprika, and garlic powder. Stir to combine.
3. Bring the mixture to a boil, then reduce heat and simmer for 20-25 minutes, or until the sweet potatoes are tender.
4. Season with salt and pepper to taste.
5. Serve the chili warm, garnished with chopped cilantro (optional).

Per serving: - Calories: 263 - Fiber: 9g - Carbs: 46g - Fats: 3g - Protein: 9g - Sugar: 8g

Snack Recipes

---

1. Popcorn with Turmeric and Black Pepper

• Total Time: 15 minutes • Serves: 2

Ingredients

- 3 cups popped popcorn
- 1 tsp turmeric
- 1/4 tsp black pepper
- 1 tbsp olive oil

Procedure

1. Pop the popcorn according to package directions.
2. In a large bowl, toss the popcorn with the olive oil, turmeric, and black pepper until evenly coated.
3. Serve immediately and enjoy!

Per serving: - Calories: 120 - Fiber: 4g - Carbs: 12g - Fats: 8g - Protein: 2g - Sugar: 0g

2. Pistachios and Dried Apricots

• Total Time: 8 minutes • Serves: 2

Ingredients

- 1/4 cup shelled pistachios
- 1/4 cup dried apricots, chopped

Procedure

1. In a small bowl, combine the pistachios and chopped dried apricots.
2. Serve immediately and enjoy!

Per serving: - Calories: 150 - Fiber: 4g - Carbs: 16g - Fats: 8g - Protein: 5g - Sugar: 12g

3. Mango Salsa with Baked Tortilla Chips

• Total Time: 30 minutes • Serves: 2

Ingredients

Salsa:
- 1 mango, diced
- 1/4 cup diced red onion
- 1 jalapeño (seeded and diced)
- 2 tbsp chopped fresh cilantro
- 1 tbsp lime juice
- 1/4 tsp salt

Tortilla Chips:
- 4 small corn tortillas (cut into wedges)
- 1 tbsp olive oil
- 1/4 tsp salt

Procedure

1. Preheat your oven to 400°F (200°C).
2. In a bowl, add all the salsa ingredients and mix well. Set aside.
3. Arrange the tortilla wedges on a baking sheet. Brush with olive oil and sprinkle with salt.
4. Bake for 8-10 minutes, flipping halfway, until crispy.
5. Serve the baked tortilla chips with the mango salsa.

Per serving: - Calories: 180 - Fiber: 5g - Carbs: 26g - Fats: 8g - Protein: 3g - Sugar: 10g

4. Roasted Chickpeas with Spices

• **Total Time: 45 minutes • Serves: 2**

Ingredients

- 1 (15 oz) can chickpeas (drained and rinsed)
- 1 tbsp olive oil
- 1 tsp ground cumin
- 1 tsp paprika
- 1/2 tsp garlic powder
- 1/4 tsp cayenne pepper
- 1/4 tsp salt

Procedure

1. Preheat your oven to 400°F (200°C).
2. Pat the chickpeas dry with a paper towel.
3. In a bowl, toss the chickpeas with the olive oil, cumin, paprika, garlic powder, cayenne pepper, and salt until evenly coated.
4. Spread the chickpeas in a single layer on a baking sheet.
5. Roast for 20-25 minutes, shaking the pan occasionally, until crispy.
6. Serve warm and enjoy!

Per serving: - Calories: 190 - Fiber: 6g - Carbs: 24g - Fats: 8g - Protein: 7g - Sugar: 2g

5. Almond Flour Muffins with Berries

• Total Time: 40 minutes • Serves: 2

Ingredients

- 1 cup almond flour
- 1/4 cup tapioca flour
- 1 tsp baking powder
- 1/4 tsp salt
- 2 eggs
- 1/4 cup honey
- 1/4 cup unsweetened almond milk
- 1/2 cup fresh or frozen berries (like blueberries or raspberries)

Procedure

1. Preheat your oven to 350°F (180°C). Grease a 6-cup muffin tin or line with paper liners.
2. In a medium bowl, whisk together the almond flour, tapioca flour, baking powder, and salt.
3. In another bowl, beat the eggs. Then, stir in the honey and almond milk.
4. Pour the wet ingredients into the dry ingredients and mix until just combined. Fold in the berries.
5. Divide the batter evenly among the prepared muffin cups.
6. Bake for 20-22 minutes, or until a toothpick inserted in the center comes out clean.
7. Allow the muffins to cool in the tin for 5 minutes before transferring to a wire rack.

Per serving: Calories: 280 - Fiber: 5g - Carbs: 26g - Fats: 16g - Protein: 8g - Sugar: 16g

6. Strawberry Banana Smoothie

• **Total Time: 10 minutes • Serves: 2**

Ingredients

- 1 cup fresh or frozen strawberries
- 1 ripe banana, peeled
- 1 cup unsweetened almond milk
- 1/2 cup plain Greek yogurt
- 1 tbsp honey (optional)

Procedure

1. Add all ingredients to your blender and blend until smooth and creamy.
2. Pour into two glasses and serve immediately.

Per serving: Calories:150 - Fiber: 4g - Carbs: 27g - Fats: 2.5g - Protein: 8g - Sugar: 16g

7. Cherry Tomato and Mozzarella Skewers

• **Total Time: 15 minutes** • **Serves: 2**

Ingredients

- 10 cherry tomatoes, halved
- 10 small mozzarella balls (or 1/2 cup diced mozzarella)
- 2 tbsp balsamic glaze
- 1 tbsp fresh basil, chopped
- Salt and pepper to taste

Procedure

1. Thread the cherry tomato halves and mozzarella balls onto skewers.
2. Drizzle the balsamic glaze over the skewers and sprinkle with chopped basil, salt, and pepper.
3. Serve immediately and enjoy!

Per serving: Calories: 120 - Fiber: 1g - Carbs: 7g - Fats: 8g - Protein: 8g - Sugar: 6g

8. Mango Slices with Chili Lime Seasoning

• Total Time: 10 minutes • Serves: 2

Ingredients

- 1 ripe mango (peeled and sliced)
- 1 tsp chili powder
- 1 tsp lime zest
- 1/4 tsp salt

Procedure

1. Arrange the mango slices on a plate.
2. In a small bowl, mix together the chili powder, lime zest, and salt.
3. Sprinkle the chili lime seasoning over the mango slices.
4. Serve immediately and enjoy!

Per serving: Calories: 60 - Fiber: 2g - Carbs: 15g - Fats: 0g - Protein: 1g - Sugar: 13g

9. Rice Cake with Avocado and Tomato

• Total Time: 15 minutes • Serves: 2

Ingredients

- 4 brown rice cakes
- 1 ripe avocado, mashed
- 1 cup cherry tomatoes, halved
- 1 tbsp fresh lemon juice
- 1 tbsp chopped fresh cilantro
- Salt and pepper to taste

Procedure

1. Spread the mashed avocado evenly over the rice cakes.
2. Top the avocado with the halved cherry tomatoes.
3. Drizzle the lemon juice over the top and sprinkle with chopped cilantro, salt, and pepper.
4. Serve immediately and enjoy!

Per serving: Calories: 190 - Fiber: 7g - Carbs: 23g - Fats: 11g - Protein: 4g - Sugar: 2g

Dessert Recipes

---

1. Baked Pears with Honey and Cinnamon

• **Total Time: 45 minutes** • **Serves: 3**

Ingredients

- 3 ripe pears (halved and cored)
- 2 tbsp honey
- 1 tsp ground cinnamon
- 1/4 cup water

Procedure

---

1. Preheat your oven to 375°F (190°C).
2. Place the pear halves in a baking dish and drizzle with honey. Sprinkle with cinnamon.
3. Pour the water into the baking dish.
4. Bake for 20-25 minutes, or until the pears are tender and easily pierced with a fork.
5. Serve warm and enjoy!

Per serving: - Calories: 120 - Fiber: 4g - Carbs: 30g - Fats: 0g - Protein: 1g - Sugar: 22g

2. Raspberry Coconut Chia Popsicles

• Total Time: 4 hours 15 minutes • Serves: 3

Ingredients

- 1 cup fresh or frozen raspberries
- 1 cup unsweetened coconut milk
- 2 tbsp chia seeds
- 1 tbsp honey (optional)

Procedure

1. In a blender, puree the raspberries until smooth.
2. In a small bowl, whisk together the coconut milk, chia seeds, and honey (optional).
3. Divide the raspberry puree and coconut-chia mixture evenly into popsicle molds.
4. Freeze for at least 4 hours, or until completely frozen.
5. Remove the popsicles from the molds and enjoy!

Per serving: - Calories: 110 - Fiber: 5g - Carbs: 12g - Fats: 6g - Protein: 2g - Sugar: 8g

3. Lemon Turmeric Coconut Bliss Balls

• **Total Time: 30 minutes** • **Serves: 3**

Ingredients

- 1 cup unsweetened shredded coconut
- 1/2 cup raw cashews
- 2 tbsp coconut oil, melted
- 1 tbsp honey
- 1 tsp ground turmeric
- 1 tsp lemon zest
- Pinch of sea salt

Procedure

1. In a food processor, blend the shredded coconut and cashews until they form a coarse meal.
2. Add the melted coconut oil, honey, turmeric, lemon zest, and salt. Blend until the mixture comes together.
3. Roll the mixture into 1-inch balls and place them on a parchment-lined baking sheet.
4. Refrigerate for at least 15 minutes before serving.

Per serving: Calories: 220 - Fiber: 3g - Carbs: 14g - Fats: 17g - Protein: 4g - Sugar: 8g

4. Dark Chocolate Avocado Mousse

• **Total Time: 45 minutes • Serves: 3**

Ingredients

- 1 ripe avocado (pitted and flesh scooped out)
- 1/4 cup unsweetened cocoa powder
- 2 tbsp honey
- 2 tbsp unsweetened almond milk
- 1 tsp vanilla extract
- Pinch of sea salt

Procedure

1. In a food processor or high-speed blender, combine the avocado, cocoa powder, honey, almond milk, vanilla, and salt. Blend until smooth and creamy.
2. Divide the mousse into serving bowls or glasses.
3. Refrigerate for at least 30 minutes before serving.

Per serving: Calories: 160 - Fiber: 5g - Carbs: 18g - Fats: 10g - Protein: 3g - Sugar: 12g

5. Sweet Potato Brownies

• **Total Time: 50 minutes • Serves: 3**

Ingredients

- 1 cup cooked and mashed sweet potato (about 1 medium sweet potato)
- 1/2 cup unsweetened applesauce
- 1/4 cup maple syrup
- 1/4 cup unsweetened cocoa powder
- 1/4 cup almond flour
- 1 tsp vanilla extract
- 1/4 tsp sea salt

Procedure

1. Preheat your oven to 350°F (175°C). Grease an 8x8-inch baking pan.
2. In a large bowl, mix together the mashed sweet potato, applesauce, maple syrup, cocoa powder, almond flour, vanilla, and salt until well combined.
3. Pour the batter into the baking pan and smooth the top.
4. Bake for 30-35 minutes, or until a toothpick inserted in the center comes out clean.
5. Allow the brownies to cool completely before cutting into squares.

Per serving: - Calories: 180 - Fiber: 4g - Carbs: 30g - Fats: 5g - Protein: 3g - Sugar: 16g

6. Almond Flour Lemon Blueberry Muffins

• **Total Time: 40 minutes** • **Serves: 2**

Ingredients

- 1 cup almond flour
- 1 tsp baking powder
- 1/4 tsp salt
- 1/4 cup honey
- 1 tbsp lemon juice
- 1 cup fresh or frozen blueberries
- 1/4 cup coconut flour
- 1/4 tsp baking soda
- 2 eggs
- 1/4 cup unsweetened almond milk
- 1 tsp lemon zest

Procedure

1. Preheat your oven to 350°F (175°C). Grease a 12-cup muffin tin or line with paper liners.
2. In a medium bowl, whisk together the almond flour, coconut flour, baking powder, baking soda, and salt.
3. In another bowl, beat the eggs. Add the honey, almond milk, lemon juice, and lemon zest, and mix well.
4. Pour the wet ingredients into the dry ingredients and stir until just combined. Fold in the blueberries.
5. Scoop the batter into the prepared muffin tin, filling each cup about 3/4 full.
6. Bake for 20-25 minutes, or until a toothpick inserted into the center comes out clean.
7. Allow the muffins to cool in the tin for 5 minutes before taking to a wire rack to cool completely.

Per serving: Calories: 220 - Fiber: 4g - Carbs: 24g - Fats: 12g - Protein: 6g - Sugar: 14g

7. Banana Almond Butter Ice Cream

• Total Time: 15 minutes • Serves: 2

Ingredients

- 2 ripe bananas, frozen
- 2 tbsp natural almond butter
- 1 tbsp unsweetened almond milk

Procedure

1. In a food processor or high-speed blender, blend the frozen bananas, almond butter, and almond milk until smooth and creamy.
2. Scoop the ice cream into serving bowls and enjoy immediately.

Per serving: Calories: 174 - Fiber: 3g - Carbs: 17g - Fats: 11g - Protein: 5g - Sugar: 10g

8. Quinoa Chocolate Chip Cookies

• Total Time: 30 minutes • Serves: 2

Ingredients

- 1/2 cup cooked quinoa, cooled
- 1/2 cup almond flour
- 1/4 cup coconut sugar
- 2 tbsp coconut oil, melted
- 1 egg
- 1 tsp vanilla extract
- 1/4 tsp baking soda
- 1/4 tsp salt
- 1/4 cup dark chocolate chips

Procedure

1. Preheat your oven to 350°F (175°C). Line a baking sheet with parchment paper.
2. In a medium bowl, combine the cooked quinoa, almond flour, coconut sugar, melted coconut oil, egg, vanilla extract, baking soda, and salt. Mix until well incorporated.
3. Fold in the dark chocolate chips.
4. Scoop tablespoon-sized balls of dough onto the prepared baking sheet, spacing them about 2 inches apart.
5. Bake for 12-15 minutes, or until the cookies are lightly golden around the edges.
6. Allow the cookies to cool on the baking sheet for 5 minutes before taking to a wire rack to cool completely.

Per serving: Calories: 156 - Fiber: 2g - Carbs: 16g - Fats: 10g - Protein: 3g - Sugar: 8g

9. Pumpkin Spice Chia Pudding

• **Total Time: 2 hours 15 minutes • Serves: 2**

Ingredients

- 1/4 cup chia seeds
- 1 cup unsweetened almond milk
- 1/4 cup pumpkin puree
- 2 tbsp maple syrup
- 1 tsp ground cinnamon
- 1/2 tsp ground ginger
- 1/4 tsp ground nutmeg

Procedure

1. In a medium bowl, whisk together the chia seeds, almond milk, pumpkin puree, maple syrup, cinnamon, ginger, and nutmeg.
2. Cover and refrigerate for at least 2 hours, or until thickened.
3. Serve chilled, garnished with additional cinnamon or a sprinkle of chopped nuts, if desired.

Per serving: - Calories: 174 - Fiber: 8g - Carbs: 22g - Fats: 8g - Protein: 5g - Sugar: 11g

10. Hazelnut Chocolate Truffles

• Total Time: 30 minutes • Serves: 2

Ingredients

- 1/2 cup raw hazelnuts
- 1/4 cup unsweetened cocoa powder
- 2 tbsp coconut oil, melted
- 2 tbsp maple syrup
- 1/4 tsp sea salt

Procedure

1. In a food processor, pulse the hazelnuts until they form a coarse flour.
2. Add the cocoa powder, melted coconut oil, maple syrup, and sea salt. Pulse until the mixture forms a smooth, sticky dough.
3. Using a small scoop or spoon, form the dough into 1-inch balls and place them on a parchment-lined baking sheet.
4. Refrigerate the truffles for at least 20 minutes to allow them to firm up.
5. Serve chilled and enjoy!

Per serving: Calories: 142 - Fiber: 2g - Carbs: 10g - Fats: 11g - Protein: 2g - Sugar: 6g

2-Week Meal Plan

WEEK 1

	BREAKFAST	LUNCH	DINNER	SNACK/DESSERT
DAY 1	PEANUT BUTTER BANANA PROTEIN SHAKE	GREEK ORZO SALAD WITH FETA	BAKED CHICKEN WITH SWEET POTATO MASH	PUMPKIN SPICE CHIA PUDDING
DAY 2	SWEET POTATO HASH WITH EGGS	BROCCOLI AND CHEDDAR SOUP	MUSHROOM AND SPINACH QUINOA RISOTTO	DARK CHOCOLATE AVOCADO MOUSSE
DAY 3	WHOLE GRAIN PANCAKES WITH MAPLE SYRUP	MEDITERRANEAN PASTA SALAD	LEMON HERB ROASTED CHICKEN THIGHS	ALMOND FLOUR MUFFINS WITH BERRIES
DAY 4	COTTAGE CHEESE WITH FRESH BERRIES	EGGPLANT PARMESAN WITH WHOLE WHEAT PASTA	ROASTED GARLIC CAULIFLOWER SOUP	BANANA ALMOND BUTTER ICE CREAM
DAY 5	BREAKFAST SALAD WITH POACHED EGG	BLACK BEAN AND CORN QUESADILLAS	BLACKENED MAHI MAHI WITH MANGO SALSA	RICE CAKE WITH AVOCADO AND TOMATO
DAY 6	BUCKWHEAT PORRIDGE WITH CINNAMON AND APPLES	FALAFEL SALAD WITH TAHINI DRESSING	LEMON DILL SHRIMP AND ASPARAGUS STIR-FRY	MANGO SALSA WITH BAKED TORTILLA CHIPS
DAY 7	MUSHROOM AND SPINACH FRITTATA	SALMON AND ASPARAGUS FOIL PACKETS	GINGER SOY GLAZED COD	CHERRY TOMATO AND MOZZARELLA SKEWERS

WEEK 2

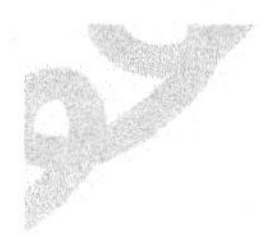
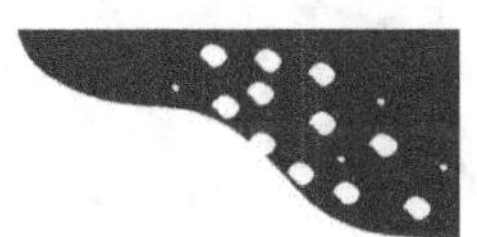

	BREAKFAST	LUNCH	DINNER	SNACK/DESSERT
DAY 1	OATMEAL WITH ALMOND BUTTER AND BANANAS	TUNA SALAD LETTUCE WRAPS	SWEET POTATO AND BLACK BEAN CHILI	QUINOA CHOCOLATE CHIP COOKIES
DAY 2	GREEN SMOOTHIE WITH KALE AND PINEAPPLE	BBQ CHICKEN AND PINEAPPLE SKEWERS	SEARED TUNA WITH CUCUMBER SALAD	RASPBERRY COCONUT CHIA POPSICLES
DAY 3	BLUEBERRY MUFFINS WITH ALMOND FLOUR	ZUCCHINI NOODLES WITH PESTO AND CHERRY TOMATOES	GREEK CHICKEN SOUVLAKI SKEWERS	HAZELNUT CHOCOLATE TRUFFLES
DAY 4	COCONUT YOGURT WITH MIXED NUTS AND SEEDS	CHICKPEA SALAD WITH LEMON DRESSING	HAWAIIAN CHICKEN PINEAPPLE BOWLS	PISTACHIOS AND DRIED APRICOTS
DAY 5	BREAKFAST WRAP WITH TURKEY BACON AND AVOCADO	LENTIL SOUP WITH SPINACH	SPAGHETTI SQUASH WITH TURKEY BOLOGNESE	ROASTED CHICKPEAS WITH SPICES
DAY 6	BREAKFAST TACOS WITH AVOCADO AND SALSA	CAULIFLOWER CRUST PIZZA WITH ARUGULA AND PROSCIUTTO	BAKED COD WITH TOMATO AND OLIVE RELISH	POPCORN WITH TURMERIC AND BLACK PEPPER
DAY 7	ACAI BOWL WITH GRANOLA AND COCONUT FLAKES	LEMON HERB CHICKEN SALAD	BUTTERNUT SQUASH AND BLACK BEAN ENCHILADAS	BAKED PEARS WITH HONEY AND CINNAMON